The Dilemma of
HIV/AIDS

The Rise, The Reign and The Ruin of
HIV/AIDS

Dr. Taiwo Akhigbe

Disclaimer

This book is intended to give accurate information on this subject matter however medical knowledge is constantly changing and information may alter. It is the responsibility of the reader of this book to consult practitioners to determine the best treatment for their patients. The author and the publisher are not liable to damages, injury or death to persons directly or indirectly by this publication.

CONTENTS

DEDICATION

In a world saturated with young people trying to find relevance with some already plagued with the deadly virus with vast majority in Sub-Saharan Africa on the brink of poverty, lack and deprivation coupled with HIV/AIDS who are fighting shame, stigma and silence to say alive in the defeat of AIDS, to them this book is gallantly dedicated, they are the unsung heroes in the final onslaught of AIDS.

PREFACE

I was striking out into new territory, I wasn't too confident, but I told people I am trying something new and I didn't know if I will make it or not, but I have the right to try.

-learned Hand

AIDS has created a worldwide emergency ....
There are no geographical safe zones and no racial exemption

- Jonathan Mann M.D World Health Organization 1987

Every day my eyes twinkle, my face feels the sweet touch of the morning sun, my ears trap fine melodies from birds, my nose sniffs the sweet aroma of the luxuriant flowers, a song of thanks for the opportunity to impact my generation through the instrumentality of creative writing.

As it is for the cheetah to sprint, the birds to sing and the cock to crow, so it is easy for me to write. In every morning devotion, in-depth study, silent moment, deep medication, thoughtful mood, is hidden a chapter to write. In the quiet chamber of my heart, I saw these chapters turned into a *masterpiece* am presenting to my generation.

I watch my generation with passion and cast-Iron concentration, they are young, fast advanced, computerized... in need, in need of the truths hidden and these must be revealed. In my heart is a passionate desire and white-hot passion to use my privileged position as a medical doctor to clarify and elucidate issues and myths surrounding *HIV/AIDS*. Hence what you are holding in your is a seed of that commitment, that is about to turn into a giant oak tree where people will get refuge by having their questions adequately answered and their hope rekindled. *HIV/AIDS* has been declared as the most devastating pandemic in human history, from the onset of the AIDS epidemic, over 70 million people have been infected with the HIV virus and 35 million deaths recorded from HIV/AIDS. At the close of 2016 36.7 million were leaving with HIV worldwide. An estimated 0.8% of adults aged 15–49 years are living with HIV globally, although the epidemic burden differs significantly between regions and countries. Currently sub-Saharan Africa remains extremely affected region with about 1 in every 25 adults (4.2%) living with HIV and accounting for nearly two-thirds of the people living with HIV globally *(Global Health Observatory Data, WHO).*

Behind every destructive influence is ignorance, Ignorance is not just the absence of knowledge but also the neglect of it. The greatest enemy of humanity is not sin or Satan but *Ignorance*. The purpose of this book is to empower and equip young and old with adequate and sound knowledge about this pandemic called *HIV/AIDS*.

The source of true freedom in life is not legislation or set of moral codes of dos and don'ts, but rather applied *knowledge*, too many people have become prisoner in their cacophony of ignorance. There is no way to walk in true freedom without shouldering its responsibility. The price of responsibility requires more time, effort and focus in acquiring this knowledge, this book is set to put an end to misinformation and half-truths associated with this subject. *Half-truths are dangerous because they imprison.* There are so many books on *HIV/AIDS* daily poured out into the information world, but this is unique because it is an impactful voice amidst secular echoes, using sound and moral principles, precept and practices to proffer solution to issues surrounding the *HIV/AIDS* pandemic. The greatest challenge in the cure of *HIV/AIDS* presently lies in it prevention hence sound moral values and precepts must be respected and strictly adhered to.

This book is also aimed at addressing millions young people plagued with the deadly *HIV/AIDS* world-wide of which vast majority are located in Sub-Saharan Africa. The future generation of young people is at stake because no one is more dangerous than a mountain man with a valley mentality; it is easier to exist in slavery than to live in freedom. Transformation begins with information; they must be sensitized to change their library, friends and influence for them to fulfill their dreams and destinies. *HIV/AIDS* Will no longer decimate future leaders of tomorrow. *We all have been victims of our past we do not have to remain prisoners of them; you can determine your future. The choice is yours and your choice will determine your destiny.*

HIV/AIDS is not a punishment from God for sexual promiscuity, neither is it a biological weapon manufactured by super-nations to decimate the ever-increasing world population. There are heinous sins dated back in the Bible days that are like those implied as one of the mode of transmission (sexual route) of *HIV,* why was *HIV/AIDS* not unleashed as punishment from God like
-The wickedness of beautiful daughters of men (Genesis 6:1-7)
- Ham viewing his father, Noah's nakedness is sexual passion called *voyeurism* (Genesis 9:22)
- The *sodomy* of Sodom and Gomorrah is homosexuality (Genesis 19:45).

- The daughters of Lot sleeping and having sexual intercourse with their father is *incestuous* (Genesis 9:33-38)

Yet God did not unleash them with a virus as punishment. We need to douse our extremist askance on *HIV* affected persons as well as people living with *HIV/AIDS (PLWHAS)* to be able to respond positively and meaningfully to them.

OUR RESPONSE

1. We need to acquire proper knowledge about *HIV/AIDS* and associated facts and help propagate and disseminate same through what so ever media. The greatest hope currently lies in its prevention.

2. Teaching sound godly values like sexual abstinence to young people and unmarried.

3. Encouraging marital fidelity among married couples.

4. More young people should be challenged to take up research interest in bio pharmaceutical if they are already in such discipline or enroll to study such disciplines.

5. We should show concern, sympathy and empathy to those people living with *HIV/AIDS*. They need our support not shame or stigma. We should point them to the true source of joy and lasting peace.

Introduction

THE MOST DEVASTATING PANDEMIC IN HUMAN HISTORY

No war on the face of the world is as destructive as the AIDS pandemic- Former US Secretary of State, Collin Powell, 2002.

The biologic clock is tolling inexorably to the time when these epidemic events are beyond society's grasp- Learned Hand.

Bogie (not real name) was a student in one of the foremost university in Nigeria. He came into the school with passion for excellence and addiction for knowledge, bubbling with dreams and visions, soon he indulged in continual pre-marital sex, he threw moral rectitude to the wind and purity to dogs. Years later, he stopped gaining weight and contacted one infection after another, finally Bogie died of HIV/*AIDS related complications.* Bogie died full of potential, ambition and destiny. He never lived full purpose in life, what a tragedy! Today Bogie if history only fit for moral lessons to future generation.

There are many Bogies that are out there living their lives on the brink of death, learn from history, those who fall to learn from history will themselves inevitably become history, beware *HIV/AIDS* is real.

History of Spread

HIV is spreading rapidly within countries and across border, it affects people regardless of gender, geographical or sexual orientation. Consequently, the world is currently inundated with AIDS epidemics diverse in their measures and the affected numbers of people. In addition, they are also different in the causative factors fueling them. Hence it has become the greatest pandemic in human history. It is estimated that over 37 million people are currently living with HIV/AIDS of which 30 percent don't know their HIV status, 76 million have become infected since the onset of this pandemic and 35 million have died from AIDS related illnesses since the onset of this pandemic. (The figures used are estimates published by UNAIDS). About 1.8 million were newly infected with HIV globally year 2016, a reduction from 2.1 million in 2015.

An estimated 25-30 million people in sub-Saharan Africa with HIV/AIDS accounts for 71% of global HIV/AIDS burden with highest infection burden from South Africa (25 percent) followed by Nigeria (13 percent) and Mozambique (six percent). Sub-Saharan Africa has become the hotbed to this pandemic with 2.4 million deaths from AIDS related complication in year 2000 which represents 80% of the global total. Hence AIDS is the major cause of death in the region. Southern

Africa has the highest infection rate than any other region in the world. In his address to the 13th international *AIDS* conference, held in Durban, South Africa in July 2000, *former South Africa president Nelson Mandela stated; we were shocked to learn that within South Africa 1 in 2, that is half, of our young people will die of AIDS. The most frightening thing is that all these infections, which statistics tell us about, the attendant human suffering... could have been, can be prevented*

In 2002 the joint united Nations programmed of *HIV/AIDS* (UNAIDS) reported: *the average life expectancy in sub-Saharan Africa is currently 47 years, without AIDS it would have been 62 years.*

In Malawi, over ten percent of the populations are infected with *HIV*. At one rural hospital, according to the Globe and Mail Newspapers; *bed occupancy is at 150 percent and the facility has lost more than 50 percent of it medical staff to AIDS.*

The plague of HIV/AIDS extends far beyond Africa continent UNAIDS estimates that some four million adults are infected with *HIV* adding that with the current disease burden, *HIV* may emerge as the largest cause of adult mortality unless adequate controlled measures fully employed.

Previously there was a rise of infection 420,000 in Eastern Europe in 1999 and 700,000 at the end of 2000 but since the advent of anti-retroviral therapy there has been a significant decline in infection rate compared to Africa. Survey conducted in six large American cities revealed a 12.3 percent rate of *HIV* infection among young gay men. Furthermore, only 29 percent of those who were *HIV* positive knew they were infected, the epidemiologist who led the survey said, *we were so disheartened to found out that, so few HIV positive men knew they were infected, that means newly infected people are transmitting the virus without knowing it. HIV/AIDS was declared the most devastating pandemic in human history in Switzerland in 2001 during the meeting of foremost AIDS researchers and scholars.*

Currently an estimated 800 000 people died in the Sub-Saharan African Region from HIV-related causes in 2015, which indicates that mortality has been halved in the past decade, this is due to accessible and affordable anti-retroviral drugs, increasing public health campaigns and government commitment.

CHAPTER ONE

GENESIS OF THE PANDEMIC

Everybody knows that pestilences have an easy way of recurring in the world; Yet somehow, we find it hard to believe in ones that crash down on our heads from a blue sky. There have been as many plagues as wars in history, yet always plagues and wars take people equally by surprise - Albert Camus, the plague (1949)

For a disease that has become the most feared killer of young and middle-aged adults, the arrival of *AIDS* on medical scene was notably inconspicuous or insidious if you will. In the late 1970's Kaposi's sarcoma, a cancerous condition normally seen in middle and older age Mediterranean men, began to appear anecdotally in young white middle class male beyond their social, economic and racial status, however, these few patients showed

1

one common denominator, a homosexual life style. A new syndrome was shortly reported in 1981 by researchers at UCLA and medical centers in New York *(Gallo RC. The AIDS virus, January 1987, P47)* The syndrome was named appropriately the Gay Related Immunodeficiency disease, but in defense to gay activism, the medical community re-named it the Acquired Immunodeficiency syndrome (David A. Noebel. The Homo-sexual Evolution, Summit Press, 1985, P. 85).

The disease appeared to represent an infection form of Immunodeficiency and soon began to surface among intravenous drug users, Haitians and blood transfusion recipient.

The species-crossing probably occurred in Equatorial Africa where the simian T-Iymphtrophic virus 111 (STLV - 111) is found innocuously in green monkeys. This appear to be very similar to, or the same virus now infecting 15% of the West Africa adult population and isolated from Senegalese prostitute. It is now named HIV2 (Initially HTLV-IV,) and a close relative of the *AIDS* virus. Testing stored blood samples reveals that *HIV* Infection was endemic in Central and Eastern Africa in the late 1950's although there is no evidence of its existence in the human population before that time. The earliest serologic documentation of *AIDS* is in East Africa around Lake Victoria bordered by Kenya, Tanzania and Uganda, (John Pekanen. *AIDS:* The plague that knows no boundaries. Reader's digest, July 1987, P52). In Southwest Uganda, for example, entire villages have been decimated by the mid 1970's, *AIDS was epidemic in Africa primarily for behavioral rather than biologic reasons*. During the post – Independence decades there have been massive population shifts in Africa with increasing urbanization, breakdown of traditional, tribal and social structure; and concurrent promiscuous sexual conduct that provide a fertile ground for an exceedingly virulent virus.

From Africa it appears to have spread to the United States and then to the Caribbean and Europe (Gallo R. The *AIDS* Virus). By the late 1970's *AIDS* had become a silent unrecognized global epidemic in one – third of a single human generation time. Any yet, having arrived the United States likely by the late 60's, nothing was heard from this pathogen until the 1980's. Why? *Nature had provided the virus, but man had to provide it mode of transmission.* Human behavior had to permit the development of sufficient reservoir of infected people whose conduct and contact would pass the virus to large numbers before themselves died from the infection. The homosexual creed and lifestyle were the ideal vector and exotic intimate behavior to a prodigious degree transported the virus throughout the United State to every corner of the globe.

The virus was isolated in 1983, since then it has claimed about 25 million lives with 13,000 new infections occurring each day. There are about 38 million people living with *HIV*, Africa bear the brunt of the epidemic with 12 million deaths already and 23 million people currently infected, there are 13 million *AIDS* orphans (as a child who is 15 years and below that has lost either mother or both parents to *HIV/AIDS*) in Africa. This is projected to increase to 30 million if current interventions are impaired.

In Nigeria *AIDS* was first reported in sexually active 13 years old girl from the western part of Nigeria. The prevalence has been on the increase. Nigeria has the second largest

HIV/AIDS epidemics in the world, second to South Africa. The nation *HIV* prevalence at the end of 2001 was 5.8%. Every day more and more people get infected. In 2002 it was estimated that 1 person die to *AIDS* every 2 minutes that is 800 Nigeria's per day, by the end of 2002, 1.4 million Nigeria's have died of *AIDS*. By the end of 2005, it was projected that another one million people will die if nothing is done (figures by National *AIDS* control programmed, Abuja March 2002)

In 2014 prevalence rate of 3.17 percent among people aged 15 to 49. Currently, it was reported in 2016 that 3.2 million people are living with HIV in a nation with over 180 million inhabitants with 2.9% adult prevalence, 220,000 new infections and 160,000 AIDS related deaths. Furthermore, 31percent adults are currently on antiretroviral therapy.

Almost over two decades later, the number of HIV cases worldwide is on the decline as a result of anti-retroviral therapy and intensive public health campaign but HIV/AIDS still a major issue in Sub-Saharan Africa. Expert suggests that the future look no less sinister, in the 45 most affected countries reports *UNAIDS*, it is projected that between 2000 and 2020, 68 million people will die prematurely because of *AIDS if no further intervention actively undertaken.* Currently some countries still practiced visa refusal or restriction for foreigners with positive HIV status.

CHAPTER TWO

AIDS: THE VIRUS AND THE DISEASE

.... I think the only co-factor is time (in determining progression of illness and death from AIDS infection) .... I think no one wants to be the first to say it -Dr. Robert Benjamin, Centers for Disease Control 1987.

We're dealing with a kind of contemporary apocalypse.

- *Stephen Lewis, UN special Envoy for HIV/AIDS in Africa*

To say that time is the only factor standing between infection and death, is to identify two hallmarks of HIV infection: the infection is an ultimately fatal condition, and there is no foreseeable cure at the present state of medical knowledge and wisdom. This is because AIDS is not only a universally fatal infection, but more fundamentally possessing a lethal genetic mutation. The infected person has

8

undergone a permanent, ongoing alteration of his inherited genetic code, which is incompatible with survival.

The two types: *HIV-1 and HIV-2,* both belong to the sub family of lentiviruses and family of retroviruses. *HIV*-1 is widely distributed all over the world while HIV–2 is mainly endemic in West Africa. However, some isolated HIV-2 infection has been reported, it is severe, and symptoms take much longer to develop, that is the incubation period is longer than in HIV-1. Also, the transmission rate of HIV-2 appears to be lower.

A foremost researcher once said; *after many, many years of peering at virus particles, through the election microscope, I have still not ceased to be amazed and excited by the precision and intricacy of design in something very, very small.*

A virus is smaller than average human cell, according to one authority, HIV is so small that *230 million (particles of HIV) would fit into the period at the end of this sentence.* Until a virus infiltrate and colonize a host cell, it cannot multiply. When *HIV* invades the body, it must contend with the body defense mechanism composed of white blood cells produced by bone marrow. Cell mediated immunity plays a major role in body defense consisting of helper T-cells which play a central role in identifying foreign invaders and assist in the destruction of these foreign invaders. HIV specifically targets these helper T-cells. Other components of body immune system are the Killer T–cells which are activated to destroy body cell that have been invaded while B-cells releases antibodies that are instrumental in the fight against infections.

Ribonucleic Acid (RNA) is the genetic blue print of HIV hence it reprograms the host cell DNA to make numerous viral copies of HIV. This is impossible except *HIV* change its own RNA so that it can be read and understood by the host cell using the virus enzyme called *reverse transcriptase*. The cells die with time after producing numerous new HIV particles which furthermore produced more particles to infect other cells.

Ultimately this lead to significant decline in the number of helper T–cells which play a central role in body immunity leading to the body susceptible to diverse diseases and opportunistic infections. Further crippling of immune system by HIV leading to *full blown AIDS*. This is plain and clear description of how HIV cripples the immune system causing further damages to the body.

Mode of transmission

There are 3 mode of *HIV* transmission

1. Sexual transmission
2. Parental transmission
3. Vertical transmission.

Sexual Transmission.

This may be through either homosexual or heterosexual intercourse. Risk of transmission is highest in rectal intercourse. Other factors which promote infectivity include very early or advanced stage of *HIV* infection, sexually transmitted disease, especially with break in the skin during intercourse.

Factors Increasing Susceptibility to Infection

1. Traumatic intercourse
2. Rectal intercourse
3. Use of vaginal muscle contracting drugs
4. Presence of concurrently genital ulcers

5. Other STDS. (Sexually Transmitted Diseases)

AIDS is largely a heterosexual disease that affect women and men, far more common in cities than rural areas. Migration and *unprotected intercourse* have been indicated as being the major or methods of spread of the disease. Indeed, *casual sex* often involving prostitutes who have no other way to earn a living; is also a major factor in *HIV* transmission.

Women who have unprotected sex with men are at higher risk of being infected than the men they have sex with, because the vagina and the anus have a large area of skin.

The virus survives better in vagina and anus than on the surface of the penis, the acid and moist environment of the vagina also gives the virus a longer life span, and finally there are more virus copies in the man's semen or sperm than there are in the vaginal fluid. Younger women have a higher risk of becoming infected with *HIV*, they are highly susceptible to infection with sexually transmitted disease during sexual intercourse. Having sexually transmitted diseases the risk of becoming infected with *HIV*. Open sores or lesion on the surface of the penis or vagina of an infected person increase the number of *HIV* virus that are released and shed during intercourse.

PARENTERAL TRANSFUSION

This is through blood, blood product and body fluid. It includes

1. Contaminated blood and blood product transfusion
2. Sharing of needles by intravenous drug abuser and users
3. Unsterilized skin piercing instrument like needles, razors

and syringes that have come in with infected blood.

4.   Sharing of blade and sharp objects for scarification and other traditional procedures.

5.   Use of unsterilized medical instrument during medical and dental procedures.

To eliminate the risk of transfusing contaminated blood, most supplies are screen for HIV antibodies and contaminated samples are withdrawn and destroyed. Blood products like factor VIII are heat treated.

VERTICAL TRANSMISSION (MOTHER TO CHILD)

This can be through

1.   Transplacental (in utero)

2.   Manipulation during birth or delivery (intrapartum) and postpartum

3.   Breast-feeding.

About 20-30% of children born to *HIV* positive mothers are infected, the rate of transmission differs from region to region according to the prevalence of disease in the area, for example in Africa with high *HIV* prevalence the rate range is 25-30%. The rate of transmission depends also on the *HIV* status of the mother whether advanced *HIV*, symptomatic or ass-symptomatic *HIV* or at the stages of *AIDS*.

Transmission through breast milk can be avoided by using alternatives milk or milk formula. The use of "zidovudine" these days has been known to reduce vertical transmission up to 45% or more. Better still in current practice, the use of "nevirapine"-a protease inhibitor at the time of delivery for mothers and its immediate application on the baby immediately after delivery has been found highly effective in stopping vertical infection.

THOSE AT RISK (HIGH RISK GROUP).

A risk activity is anything that makes it possible for the virus to pass from one person to another. *HIV* does not discriminate among ethnic group, age, gender, rich or poor, educated or not educated, cities, villages, everybody is vulnerable to *HIV*. Risky behaviors are

1. People with multiple sexual partners i.e. sexually promiscuous individual.
2. Commercial sex workers and their clients
3. Male homosexuals
4. Long distance truck drivers
5. Mobile police men
6. Intravenous drug abusers and users.
7. Multiple transfusion recipients for example hemophiliac and sicklers.
8. Bar tenders
9. Bisexual males.

WAYS IN WHICH HIV IS NOT TRANSMITTED

Casual and social contact do not spread *HIV*

1. Touching, hugging or shaking of hands

2. Sharing of food, utensils, towels, and toilet swimming pool.

3. Staying in the same room

4. Peck on the cheek

5. Light kissing

6. Sneezing or coughing

7. Insect or animal bite.

SURVIVAL DURATION OF THE VIRUS OUTSIDE THE BODY.

HIV can survive outside the human body in a wet environment for seven day and in a dry environment for three days. (Manual on *HIV/AIDS* by WHARC, Nigeria).

NATURAL HISTORY

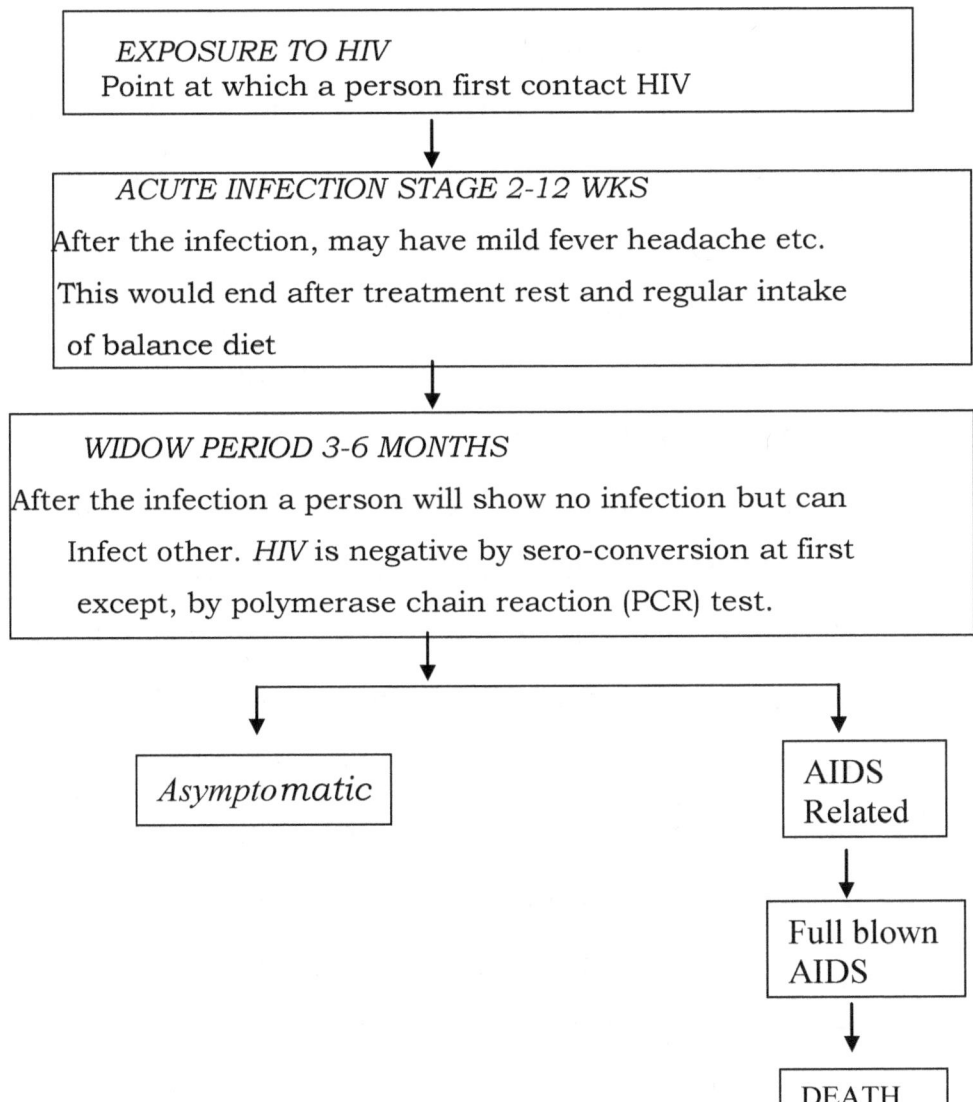

EXPOSURE TO HIV
Point at which a person first contact HIV

↓

ACUTE INFECTION STAGE 2-12 WKS
After the infection, may have mild fever headache etc.
This would end after treatment rest and regular intake
of balance diet

↓

WIDOW PERIOD 3-6 MONTHS
After the infection a person will show no infection but can
Infect other. HIV is negative by sero-conversion at first
except, by polymerase chain reaction (PCR) test.

Asymptomatic

AIDS Related

↓

Full blown AIDS

↓

DEATH

COURSE OF HIV INFECTION.

Even though the course of *HIV* infection may vary among individual patients, there is still however a common pattern recognized. Following exposure, there is a widespread dissemination of the virus in the peripheral blood (viremia) and a marked decrease in the T4 cell count. As a result of viremia, there is a definite humoral and cellular immune response (seroconversion). This takes about 3-17 weeks on the average, but may take longer period of months, after which detectable antibodies can be found in the blood. Subsequently, a period of clinical latency ensues which could last 5-10 years or longer. During this incubation period, the patient remains asymptomatic, clinical disease may set in if triggered by certain factors like the presence of other sexually transmitted infections and high-risk sexual behaviors. The onset of symptoms is also accompanied by changes in cell mediated immune response, there is a progressive decrease in number of CD4 cells, which result in a deteriorating immune status. At this point opportunistic infections set in and death may follow in two to five years. This is the final stage know as *AIDS*, characterized by the present of one or two opportunistic infection and a complete shot down of the immune system.

Major Symptoms of AIDS

1. Persistent or recurrent fever lasting up to one month
2. Chronic diarrhea lasting up to one month
3. Weight loss of at least ten percent of normal weight in the last one month.
4. Chronic cough lasting up to one month

Minor Symptoms

1. White patches in the mouth and throat (oral and   pharyngeal thrush)

2. Persistent tiredness

3. Swelling of the glands in the armpit, neck or groin, itchy skin rashes

4. Sores in the body

HIV Clinical Examination

Central Nervous System (CNS)

- CNS Lymphoma

-Focal features

EYES

-      Retinitis

FACE

-      Skin Lesions

-      Seborrhoeic dermatitis

-      Mucocutaneous herpes simplex

-      Kaposis Sarcoma

-      Molluscum Contagiasum

- Fat loss (antiretroviral drug-induced)

- Gingivitis
- Candidiasis
- Oral hairy leucoplakia
- Kaposi sarcoma

NECK, AXILLAE
- Lymphadenopathy

ABDOMEN
- Hepatosplenomegaly
- Fat redistribution (antiretroviral drug-induced)

LIMBS
Fat gain (anti- retroviral drug-induced)

PERIPHERAL NERVES
- Numbness

-    Absent reflexes

ANOGENTAL REGION

-    Rashes

-    Mucocutaneous herpes simplex

-    Sexually transmitted infection

OBSERVATION

-    Breathlessness

-    Weight loss

-    Kaposi sarcoma

-    Lipodystrophy

LABORATORY TESTS AVAILABLE

There are several tests available including ELISA tests and rapid test for confirmation. The broad principle of all tests is to detect serum antibodies produced by the body after exposure, some tests however detect the presence of antigen and they are:

1.   *Enzyme Linked immunosorbent Assay (ELISA)* is the most frequently used method for screening. However, in communities with limited laboratory facilities, rapid tests are useful and simple to use.

2.   There are several commercial rapid tests kits available from, various pharmaceutical companies.

3.   Supplemental test includes western blot- immunofluorescence and solid phase radio-immunoassay

4.   One of the most current and sophisticated methodology   today   in research is PCR and in situ hybridation. They are molecular biological method employing the analysis of the virus genetic material, RNA. They are very sensitive method which are useful in the early detection of *HIV* infection. The viral antigen can be detected long before seroconversion. Whichever test is used, all screening must   be   confirmed   with   a

supplemental test like western blot, which is more specific, confirmation is important to avoid false positive result, especially here in Africa where lots of other infection are common. Antibodies formed from other previous tropical disease can cross-react in *HIV* screening tests to give a false test result. Note that a negative HIV test result does not always mean, non-infection. It could mean that the blood sample could have been taken during the window period when no detectable antibodies have been formed. Confirmation of screened samples can also be ascertained using two or three screening rapid test of different principles.

MANAGEMENT OF HIV/AIDS

Management can be approached in several ways including

    1.   Treatments of opportunistic infection

2. Relief of respiratory distress, central nervous disorders, diarrhea, malnutrition and dehydrations.
3. Specific anti- retroviral drug therapy.

SPECIAL CONSIDERATION OF CASUAL TRANSMISSION.

Casual transmission lacks any specific definable meaning, it could be referred to a precise type and degree of inter personal conduct, it might be a useful analytical tool. Emanating from this undefined concept is litany of statements to the effect that *casual contact* is incapable of spreading *HIV* infection. *AIDS* cannot be spread by *casual contact* is an often-repeated declaration which has little meaning and falsely reassuring. For example, in the April 9, 1987 issue of the Western Medical Journal (*Flynn NM, et al. Absence of HIV antibody among dental professionals*

27

expose to infected patient) a group of Francisco investigators concluded that casual transmission was not possible based on the absence of demonstrable infection among dentist treating (and expose to salve and blood from) *AIDS* patient in their sampled cohort.

On the other hand, the CDC reported in the February 28, 1986 issue of JAMA the case of a young mother infected by her newborn infant. The infants incurred infection via transfusion and were subsequently cared for by the mother who two years later was found to be infected as a result of exposure to be child's fluids and secretions. This occurred despite inability to culture the virus from the seropositive child. These two reports emphasized the divergent conclusion derived from roughly similar type of HIV exposure, in neither case was there intimate sexual contact or direct blood transfer of infected body fluids demonstrated. It is for this reason that the phrase *casual contact* should be discarded. In it stead it must be emphasized that for infection to occur, all that need transpire is the introduction of virtually any body fluids with a sufficient viral concentration from an infected person to an uninfected person in some manner and this occur with common types of contact.

It is based on this premise for example that surgeon at UCLA medical center routinely wear goggles while operating on known *HIV* infected patients (Robinson G surgery in patient with *AIDS*, Arch surg. Feb 1987, Vol 122, p 175). The point is that some modes of contact facilitate this infection process more easily than others. However categorical statement exercising the possibility of *HIV* transmission beyond the confines of intercourse and direct viral inoculation (transfusion, needle-sharing among drug addicts, organ transplants, and perinatal infection) are medically insupportable and irresponsibly misleading. I rest my case.

INSECT TRANSMISSION

Many viral illnesses are known to be transmitted by insect. This is not meant to imply that this occurs with *AIDS*, but only that *AIDS* seemingly poses no categorical exception to this well recognized fact.

Virus (including retroviruses like *AIDS*) are propagated generally in two ways by insects. In some insects, the virus becomes biologically integrated into the bug indefinitely, and is excreted during further blood sucking meals. The less common mode of infection via insects if from contamination of mouth parts, which then inject viral particles into the next host – so called mechanical transmission. This incidentally occurs with *enquine (horse) infectious anemia* via flies whose genetic make-up is very similar to *HIV.*

Five hundred arboviruses (those incorporated into and transmitted by insect vectors) are now identified ... *About a hundred of which are associated with human being.*

Some concern is raised by the knowledge that *HIV* virus in infected people multiplies in the superficial skin tissue, where insects feed. This finding indicates that live virus is at least accessible to biting insects and skin possesses specific target cells receptive to *HIV* infection, macrophages (Langerhans cells) and T4 Lymphocytes, both of which carry the CD4 receptor, which facilitates infection with the *AIDS* virus.

Dr. Shope of the Yale Arbovirus unit, states *there are retroviruses in horses transmitted by biting flies. The hypothesis that AIDS mighty be transmitted by flies or other insects is perfectly logical and within the realm of possibility, I don't think people should believe it until it is proven, and if it is not proven we should not believe it. I don't think we can explain all the cases of AIDS.*

The United States' Center for Disease Control have published no relevant insect studies that will put this question to rest, despite many years of opportunity to do so. Further research is awaited to answer this question beyond reasonable doubt. But currently HIV/AIDS cannot be transmitted through insect bite.

CHAPTER 3

AIDS SPREADS IN AFRICA: FACTS AND FACTORS

We are dealing with a kind of contemporary apocalypse

- Stephen Lewis UN special envoy for HIV/AIDS in Africa.

The young elite represents Africa's post-independence generation to come to power. In several capitals they are already infected, heavily infected, and will die in increasing numbers. The political, social and economic and psychological impact of this gathering death march cannot be underestimated

-John pekkanen (AIDS: The plague that knows no boundaries, Reader's Digest, June 1987, P.53)

Those words typify the burden of the *AIDS* epidemic in sub-Saharan Africa which is the region of the world that is mostly affected by

33

HIV /AIDS. In this region about 26.6 million people are living with *HIV/AIDS* and approximately 3.2 million new infections occurred in 2003. The epidemic has claimed the lives of an estimated 2.3 million Africa with ten million young people and over eleven million people orphaned by AIDS.

The scale of the epidemic is currently influenced by accessibility and affordability anti-retroviral therapy which has led to significant decline in the AIDS death toll. The spread of HIV/AIDS is also on the decline but in most rural areas this may be different.

Several factors are involved in the spread of *HIV/AIDS* which in turn has exacerbated other problems. The *AIDS* epidemics in Africa are due to the following:

MORAL STANDARD

The primary and commonest means of HIV infection is sexual contact or route; moral standard deficiency including promiscuity and multiple sexual partners evidently promotes the spread of HIV/AIDS especially in developing or third- world countries who are economically and informationally disadvantaged. Sexual abstinence among the unmarried and faithfulness on the part of the married should be advised and encouraged. To simply warn young people to abstain from sex will not work writes Francous Dufour in the star newspaper of Johannesburg, South Africa *they are bombarded daily with sexual image of what they should look like and how they should behave.*

Current analysis and survey on the sexual conduct of young people for example a survey indicated that about a third of youths between the ages of 12 and 17 had engaged in sexual intercourse. This may be due to the fact that young people are daily bombarded with sexually explicit images, dressing, music, videos and programs punctuated with sexual innuendos, it's a sexually filled and driven world. This has encouraged to a certain extent rape incidence especially in cases where there is a myth that an HIV carrier who rapes a virgin will be cured as reported in some parts of South Africa, in this clime, the rape of children is on the increase. People should be empowered with adequate and balanced information about *HIV/AIDS*.

SEXUALLY TRANSMITTED DISEASE (STD)

There is a high rate of STD in Africa associated with behavior and practices that put people at risks of sexually transmitted disease and ultimately promotes HIV spread like multiple sexual partners, use of drugs that influence decision making ability resulting in poor sexual judgement and moral indiscipline.

POVERTY

Many countries in Africa are battling with poverty and this creates a favorable climate for the spread of *AIDS*. Sub-Saharan Africa has the lowest gross domestic product (GDP) in the world with over 60% leaving on less than one US dollar per day. They lack not only finance but skills, assets and basic amenities hence some of them engage in risky behaviors like commercial sex work and full-time prostitution to make ends meet. Poverty also include deprivation leading malnutrition and poor medical services. Sex and child trafficking are largely due to extreme poverty.

IGNORANCE AND MISINFORMATION

Ignorance is still a significant risk factor in the spread of HIV/AIDS in Sub-Saharan Africa. Also, misinformation about HIV/AIDS is the breeding ground for stigmatization which has led to many people declining HIV screening for fear of been denied of employment opportunities, housing benefits or visa refusal to foreign countries if HIV positive. The most devastating is fear of been shunned and isolated by friends and colleagues, many end up lonely and lapsed into depression and other mental illness because of chronic rejection from friends, families and love ones once their HIV status is revealed. Some have committed suicide and others harboring suicidal ideation because of fear of stigmatization of HIV/AIDS. As a result of stigmatized people living with HIV/AIDS, right and adequate information dissemination must be at the heart of HIV/AIDS campaigns in Africa.

Young people aged 15-24 are mostly hit by HIV/AIDS because they lacked adequate information or have misinformation of how they can protect themselves and what to do if HIV positive.

CULTURE

Culture is a significant determinant of HIV/AIDS spread in Africa especially in rural communities and settlement where traditional practices like scarification, female genital mutilation and male circumcision are common place, these are risk factors for HIV transmission no matter how low the statistics may be. Some cultural beliefs still ascribe HIV/AIDS to witchcraft hence they seek healing from witchdoctors for AIDS related illness and complication.

Also, in some rural communities women are not permitted to demand sexual accountability in extramarital affairs from their partner, this is seen as a taboos especially in cultural setting that treat women like second class citizen.

POOR MEDICAL FACILITIES

In Sub-Saharan Africa where HIV/AIDS infection rate is much, there has been a corresponding dearth or scarcity of standard medical facilities for HIV screening, CD4 count estimation and further investigation of AIDS related illness or complications. The available ones are either obsolete or overstretched. Furthermore, increasing cases of HIV/AIDS without corresponding staff or manpower to attend to them leading to substandard medical services which negatively impact on patients and service outcome.

CHAPTER 4

HIV/AIDS AND YOUNG PEOPLE

Global success in combating HIV/ AIDS must be measured by its impact on our children and young people. Are they getting the information they need to protect themselves from HIV? Are girls being empowered to take charge of their sexuality? Are infants safe from the disease, and are children orphaned by AIDS being raised in loving supportive environments? These are the hard questions we need to be asking. These are the yardsticks for measuring our leaders. We cannot let another generation be devastated by AIDS

--- Carol Bellamy, Ex-executive Director, UNICEF.

One of the ways to control or end the spread of HIV/AIDS is to focus on young people because AIDS is the leading cause of death of young people aged 10 and 24 (as defined by WHO) in

Sub-Saharan Africa. Sexual route or unprotected sex is the commonest route of transmission in young people. Young people are vulnerable because they are sexually active, they are influence by drugs and peer pressure, they lack adequate information of how to protect themselves and those in extreme poverty are sexually exploited. Hence our greatest hope in the defeat of AIDS lies in prompt, strategic and huge public intervention of this age group, this I believe will make a significant impact in the prevention of HIV/AIDS pandemic. Unfortunately, young people are always sidelined in planning and execution of AIDS intervention programs, their voices and suggestions are not heard or taken on board. They are obviously absent in most HIV/AIDS summit, conferences and workshops, they must be at the epicenter of this campaign because they are the key to the prevention of the HIV/AIDS pandemic.

The quality of information determines the quality of choices and decisions, at the center of HIV spread in young people is ignorance and misinformation. Those young people who are ignorant about *HIV* often do not protect themselves because they lack the skill, the support or means to adopt safe behaviors, it is imperative to pay due attention to vulnerable young people.

Focused and goal directed sex education will help in reducing risk behaviors and avoid steps that lead to unprotected sex or rape; encourage sexual abstinence and modelled to young people pathway to sexual integrity. Investment in HIV knowledge by young people will certainly lead to a decline in infection rate. HIV/AIDS information clinic should empower young people to take responsibility of their sexual health by going for voluntary HIV screening to know their status and commence treatment if positive or reinforce and maintained sexual abstinence if negative.

Youth behavioral intervention with use of social media can reach larger population of young people because young people are the largest users of internet and social media worldwide even currently in developing nations, this medium can be used as a template or platform to support young people leaving with HIV/AIDS.

CHAPTER 5

YOUNG PEOPLE AND PREMARITAL SEX

Young people need adult assistance to deal with the thought, feeling and experience that accompany physical maturity...

Evidence from around the world has clearly shown that providing information and building skills on human sexuality and human relationship to avert health problem and create more mature and responsible attitude – Dr. Gro Harem Brundtlan, Ex Director General World Health Organization.

We boast to young people about our great breakthrough in preventing pregnancy and treating venereal disease disregarding the most reliable and specific, the least expensive and least toxic prevention of both gestation and venereal disease, the ancient, honorable and even healthy state of virginity- Dr. Richard Lee (in Yale Journal of Biology and Medicine)

This is the age of *no absolutes* but *more relatives* hence the tendency to have liberty without restriction and the end result is anarchy. Many young people see rules about moral conduct and standard as restricting, funny or crazy. They think they will find fulfillment if left alone. Premarital sex is an abomination to moral standard, a disgrace to purify and a shame to chastity.

Sexual activity begins in adolescent for majority of people. But in many countries unmarried girls and boys are sexual active before the age of 15. Recent survey of boys 15 to 19 in Brazil, Hungary and Kenya, for example showed that more than a quarter reported having sex before they were 15. Premarital sex is a significant risk factor of *HIV/AIDS transmission.*

There are two sets of young people who fall into premarital sex.

1. The first set lack temperance (control of passion and moderation of desire). They have wrong exposure.

2. The ignorant that is unaware of the steps that could lead to premarital sex.

In the article *the first love Affair* John B. Thompson said *in the first love affairs, the average youngster is not hunting a life mate. It is (only) giving valid expression to normal impulses to grow.* This is the reason why young people fall in and out of love so often with bout of premarital sex at it wake before they eventually settle down.

FIVE TRUTHS ABOUT SEX (PREMARITAL)

1. Sex may be physical, but it involves the whole body (1 Corinthians 6; 18)

2. Premarital sex is a grievous sin (I Corinthians 6; 13)

3. There is cleaving of the soul (soul-ties) during sexual intercourse, the experience is difficult to forget (Gen 34)

4. Sex does not just happen; it is a product of little decisions made.

5. Unless you are ready for fidelity and commitment, then you are not ready for parenthood, sex can result to pregnancy.

SEX TRAP

The bait that Satan uses for sex trap is *our passion*, our complex chemical and hormonal system are easily stimulated or affected by outside factor and they can ignite incredible fires of passion and motivation in young people. Human passion, properly motivated can birth nations, win wars, defy death, overcome impossible obstacle and seal marriage with unbreakable devotion, improperly motivated can destroy nations, ignite devastating wars, bring violent death, make the smallest obstacle impossible, and destroy the best of marriage through callous betrayal, selfishness and rejection.

Where have you being looking lately? Are your eyes and desire wondering to *forbidden field*, are you at your workplace on Mondays or all week long while gazing at the woman who keep watching you week after week with illicit hunger, watch out? Your passion is on fire and you are about to fall into Satan bait.

Experts have said that women are the most powerful creatures that can control men through the instrumentality of sex. The former president of America Bill Clinton was once a victim of sexual power. Sex has wounded the lives of many great and renowned men.

For those of us who know classical history it was said that when *Pericle* went to war as a leader of Athens. It was because of lateria (first grade prostitute), Asparia whom he wanted to satisfy. Doctors have been alleged to treat patient for sex in lieu of money. Sex has been known to secure employment, win contracts for women. For the men, don't forget, *the last but-stop to gate of hell is the backside of a strange woman (proverbs 7; 26, 27).*

5 ROADS THAT LEAD TO SEX TRAPS

1. A fascination with and compulsive desire for the   forbidden just like Eve in the Garden of Eden. Eve ignored the blessing of the paradise in her fascination for the forbidden.
2. Compulsive need for ego fulfillment, even if the thing that fulfils is illegal or illicit.
3. The world increasing pressure on young girls through   media and advertising to

look alluring, sexy and attractive to the opposite sex. You are in serious trouble if your personal identity is linked to your personal success in generating sexual appeal.

4. The lie that says you deserve to have some fun and reward yourself.

5. The flesh continual craving for variety, (King Solomon, 1kings 11: 14)

VICTIMS OF SEX TRAP

It is the bait that seals your fate, the most effective trap in the natural world uses bait. Bait is carefully prepared deceit, it is death on the stick, an enticement engineered to speak to corresponding hunger or appetite, it leads one from freedom to bondage. It looks good and smells nice, but it is connected to deadly trap. The victims' sex traps are young people who cannot understand and manage their passion (sexuality).

FIVE THINGS THAT HAPPEN WHEN YOU ENGAGE IN PREMARITAL SEX

1. You sin against your body
2. You sin against person you had premarital sex with
3. You enter spiritual realm of soul tie
4. You are under the influence of spiritual harlotry
5. It is an act of satanic worship hence you become an instrument of the devil.

BENEFITS OF ABSTINENCE FROM PREMARITAL SEX

I.   Medical benefits
II. Emotional benefits
III. Relational benefits
IV. Personal benefits

MEDICAL BENEFITS

1. Protection from sexual transmitted infection like *HIV\AIDS*, gonorrhea, syphilis etc.
2. Free from unwanted pregnancy
3. Free from abortions and it's complication

EMOTIONAL BENEFITS

1. Protection from sexual addiction
2. Protection from early marriage, it consequences and complications
3. Protection from bad relationship
4. Free from guilt
5. Free from deep scar
6. Protection from misleading feeling
7. Helps in developing respect and integrity

RELATIONAL BENEFIT

1. It enhances true communication in relationship

2. It helps in building patience and self-control

3. It helps in developing positive principle of marital relationship.

4. Abstinence provides you one of the greatest gifts in relationship

VIRGINITY

PERSONAL BENEFITS

1. Abstinence helps to increase your self esteem

2. It can be a true test of love in relationship.

HOW TO WALK IN SEXUAL INTEGRITY

1. Find your fulfillment in Christ

2. Set boundaries in your speech, your actions and your appearance

3. Avoid bad companies, illicit literatures and movies, bad places and bad music.

YOUNG PEOPLE AND SEXUALITY

We seem to live in a *sex saturated world* nothing seems to arrest their interest unless it is imbued with *sexual passion* and inclination. Today, television, home video, music interest, advertorial and programs are inundated with full menu of sexual delights, flaunting premarital and extramarital sex, oh! What a generation in disarray.

Sexuality spans through the entire you, single or married, it is good and normal but must exercise temperance that is control of passion and moderation of desire.

Lust has been described by Garry Collins as passion of sexuality. This is what generally gives birth to sex (fornication) and extramarital sex (adultery). Lust is not just looking at the opposite sex but looking with a desire to have him or her. It is an evil desire that sees the opposite sex as sex symbols.

TEN REASONS FOR SEXUAL TEMPTATION

1. We live in a sex saturated world: There is an undue publicity of sex in our society, the social media, live stream video and internet adverts and music oozes out a catalogue of sexual menu.

2. Changing Standards of Sexual Menu: premarital sex used to be a taboo and virginity virtue the reverse is the case today.

3. Inappropriate sex education: from friends (peers), Films, novels and magazines. These sources of ideas are warped and unbalanced.

4. Illicit dressing: The type of dressing that is suggestive and provocative.

5. Curiosity: The undue publicity on sex creates curiosity, which the young people want to experience.

6. Peer pressure: Very often young are terribly misinformed by their peers like severity of pimples on the girl's face is because she is not having sex; Painful menstruation (dysmenorrhea) is because she has not had sex; Failing to start early sex will result in organ dysfunction and inability for sexual satisfaction when married.

7. Seduction

8. Satanic manipulation; Ephesians 6:10-13, the devil is desperate to spoil your testimony.

9. Personal internal conflict: Emotional battle against loneliness.

10.   Ignorance of the outcome of premarital sex.

PRECAUTION

1. Recognized that sexual drive is human, don't feel indifferent, control it.

2. Determine and choose the sexual limits you can handle, don't go beyond the boundary, and be careful.

3. Be honest about your strength and weakness, don't   pretend

4. Avoid places, and properties that will lead you to sexual   sins.

5. Have established standard before you enter a relationship.

6. Maintain your personal relationship with Jesus.

7. Depend and draw strength from the Holy Spirit.

8. Discern substances, signs of attraction that stimulate you and avoid them.

9. Share your struggles with spiritually sound people for   godly counsel.

10.   Avoid fanaticizing about sex.

CHOOSE ABSTINENCE.

This is God's choice on principle of sexuality, if you've fallen into sexual sin be quick to repent and confess it, if you delay, the feeling will overwhelm you.

CHAPTER 6

PREGNANCY AND HIV/AIDS

The womb of a generation should be preserved because it is the pathway of great men and women yet unborn, protect future destinies from this virus – Dr. Taiwo Akhigbe

A woman who is infected with *HIV* can still become pregnant and have a baby. However, if a woman's partner is not infected, he is at high risk of contracting the virus if they have unprotected sex. An *HIV* positive woman is treated the same way as any pregnant woman, but extra precautionary measures is taken during pregnancy and to reduce the chances of the fetus of anyone else becoming infected, however labor is not advised.

Research shows that about one in six babies born to an infected mother will have the virus. A woman who has recently been infected or who has *AIDS* is more likely to have an infected baby.

Transmission rates can be significantly reduced through treatment with drugs called antiretrovirals, which reduce the amount of virus in the blood (viral load). They are usually given towards the end of pregnancy, as from the 8th month. Without the use of antiretroviral drugs, a baby delivered through caesarean section will have a risk of contracting *HIV*. A woman who is *HIV* positive and pregnant should discuss her option with her doctor. Breast-feeding doubles the risk of transmission. Where safe alternatives, to breast milk exist, it is recommended that an HIV positive woman should not breast-feed her baby. This can be emotionally difficult and a woman in this situation should be supported. Some substitutes for breast-feeding are:

-Breast milk from an uninfected relative

-Breast milk from surrogate mothers who are not infected

-Infant formula like SMA

VERTICAL TRANSMISSION OF HIV/AIDS

A large pool of pregnant women exists for the propagation and transmission of the infected to these infants and probably to their *HIV* negative spouses as neither husband nor their infants could safely be protected in the absence of voluntary counseling and confidential or routine testing for *HIV*, antiretroviral therapy, alternative feeding formulae and protective coitus.

Vertical transmission of *HIV* can occur during pregnancy, labor, delivery and puerperium.

It can be transmitted during the following:

1. Ante partum hemorrhage
2. Co-infection e.g. *HIV* + Hepatitis B
3. Fetal prematurity
4. Virulence of the organism

5. Breast-feeding.

6. Intrapartum factors that increase the risks of vertical transmission

7. Rupture of membrane. (Greater than four hours)

8. Prolonged labor

9. Chorioamniotis

10. Instrumental delivery (vacuum is worse than forceps)

11. Episiotomy.

For women on antiretroviral drugs early enough whose viral load is less than 1000 per ml the risk of vertical transmission is less than 2%, which make no difference to the one by caesarean section.

The factors that may enhance mother to child (vertical) transmission are:

1. Maternal immunological status

2. Maternal nutritional status

3. Clinical status

4. Behavioral factors such as intravenous drug use.

5. Multiple sexual partners

6. Blood transfusion (of infected blood)

EFFECTS OF HIV ON PREGNANCY

Through it is generally reported that *HIV* has little effect on pregnancy outcome and complication in the developed countries than developing countries. This may be due to multiple factors of base line immunity of the women, adequate antenatal care, early diagnosis and antiretroviral therapy and marked reduction in viral load.

In poor and sub-Saharan Africa countries adverse effects are quite common due to the following:

1. Higher spontaneous abortion

2. Intrauterine growth restriction

3. Stillbirth

4. Urinary tract infection and other opportunistic infections.

5. Premature delivery

6. Low birth weight

7. Malaria infestation tends to be higher in *HIV* positive women.

MANAGEMENT OF HIV POSITIVE PREGNANT WOMEN

1. Voluntary testing and counseling

2. Determination of current status

3. Early antenatal looking

4. Early antenatal intervention.

CHAPTER 7

CONDOM CAN FAIL

The possible consequences of condom failure are serious enough and the likelihood of failure sufficiently high that condom use by risk groups should not be described as safe sex

- Kelly J. St Lawrence University of Mississippi medical center.

And remember boys, don't be no dunce, only use that condom once

- The condom Rag (foolish song)

The lyrics from the above song was a result of a $ 450,000 Illinois state sponsored campaign to educate the populace and performed under the auspices of the Illinois public health department on April 29, 1987, Governor James R. Thompson observed, *it's outrageous, everyone will think we are Lunatics.* The *Rag* continues, *pardon the pun, it's in the bag. All*

66

you got to do is the condom rag; Governor Thompson promptly expunged further performances stating; *what about children passing by? Is that the kind of songs you want to listen to with your children? People will think we have taken leave of our senses* (condom Rag yanked from Illinois Anti-*AIDS* campaign. American Medical News, 1ˢᵗ May 1987).

Uninformed people believed that condoms have become the talisman against *AIDS*, despite mounting evidence about their ineffectiveness in preventing *HIV* transmission accompanied by well published statement to this effect. Thus, the centers for disease control comments in October 1987: *However, even when condoms are properly used for each act of sex intercourse, infected parties and their sexual partners should fully understand that some risks of infection remain.*

And this risk of fatal infection is quantifiably significant. A paper by Dr. Fischl of the University of Miami reports a substantial failure rate for *AIDS* (JAMA 2nd Feb. 1987, 257: 447-9). Among hetero-sexual couples studied using condoms in which one partner was infected, 10% of the uninfected partners became infected. The figure increased to 30% with in the year.

A government inspection program found that condoms from 1 of every 5 batches tested, leaked when filled water. This led to a large-scale government recall (*condom makers issue recall over leaky product*. Los Angeles Herald Examiner, 20 June 1987).

A report subsequently published by the department of Health and Human services conclusion after reviewing the available data from many sources; *there are no chemical (human) data supporting the value of condoms in preventing the spread of a range of disease including... human immunodeficiency virus (HIV), the precursor of AIDS.* Condoms even have an ample failure rate in preventing pregnancy despite a substantial boost from nature during any monthly cycle there are only a few fertile days during which conception is possible, on the other hand, *AIDS* virus can be transmitted every day of the month and the virus is 30 times smaller than the human sperm, posing a much more formidable challenge to any barrier.

13-15% of women whose male partners use condoms as the sole method of contraception became pregnant within one year - Kelly J, et al, cautions about condoms Lancet. 7 Feb 1987, p 323.

This prompts Jeffrey Kelly of the University of Mississippi medical center, to predict... *the likelihood that the homosexual individual's partner will be HIV infected is substantial. Given the failure rate of condoms in family planning, homosexual who practice anal intercourse will still be at the risk of HIV exposure (infection) even if they use condoms.*

One is unforgivably native and uninformed to believe that more education in the use of condoms is the panacea to *HIV/AIDS* transmission. Condoms protect poorly against pregnancy and while, if at all, against *AIDS* with repeated exposure.

CHAPTER 8

VACCINES AND CURE

The (AIDS) Infection will become self-sustaining, ubiquitous and perpetual--- William T O'Connor MD, April 1987.

Without a vaccine or cure on the near horizon-- California medical Association, March 1987.

The *AIDS* Virus presents medical researchers with formidable obstacles and no ready solutions currently. Effective vaccines have never been developed for any of the family of retroviruses (of which *AIDS* is a member) in over eighty years of research. The current impasse in vaccine development for *HIV* does not stem simply from its recent emergence as a lethal pathogen, nevertheless, the acquaintance with *AIDS* is brief, and the inherent problems are long standing.

No natural immunity develops to this disease. Characterizing the core of this dilemma is the well reported fact that antibody production (the therapeutic gate of vaccines) has had no demonstrably protective effect against the inexorable progression to illness and death in those naturally infected. Soon after infection with HIV, antibody production is brisk and high as are virus concentrations in various body fluid. Both coexist in high concentration for several years and then slowly fall as the T4 cell population inexorably declines with advancing illness and approaching death. As Dr Francis of the CDC has noted *indeed, one of the most remarkable aspects of HIV is it propensity for producing a persistent viremic (carrier) state in a high proportion of infected people despite the presence of antibody* (Francis DC et al. The prevention of *AIDS* in the United States. JAMA 13 March 1987, vol. 257, No10.)

The impotence of naturally induce antibodies is very likely in large part due to the exceedingly high mutation rate of the virus resulting in multiple distinct antigenic strains in a single infected person: *HIV₁* (and now *HIV₂*) is an incredibly mutagenic virus. The problem is, it changes its outer protein coat (the substance by which our immune system recognizes it and mounts a defensive antibody responses) exceedingly rapidly. This results in multiple different and continually changing antigenic strains systems in a single infected person which the immune system is incapable of responding to. Infact, the National Cancer Institute in America has already Isolated 200 antigenically distinct strains from *AIDS* patients base on this observation, development of an effective vaccine is theoretically impossible. This mutability has critical implications, as Dr Luc Montagnier has noted *the potential for genetic variations is perhaps the greatest danger in future of the AIDS epidemic. It will make it difficult to design efficient vaccines protective against all strains, and a further change of the virus in it tropism (ability to infect different types of cells), and ways of transmission cannot be excluded* (Martin M et al, international conference on *AIDS* 14 17 April 1985 Atlanta).

The Virus is so highly changeable because of its genetic capabilities that many variant forms are found in the same infected person. This prompts from Dr Malcom Martin, chief of the laboratory of molecular microbiology in the infectious diseases institute to posit; *in contrast to other retroviruses, such as HTLV₁ and HTLV₂, this virus is very heterogeneous in genomic (gene) structure; its five or six genes are very unstable. The data from our laboratory and others suggest that there isn't a single virus entity Isolated from a given person. The same person can harbor multiple forms of the virus.*

This problem was predicted by Dr J. Seale, a renowned British gynecologist;

The almost unlimited varieties of antigenic strains of lentiviruses, (the family of which AIDS belongs) produced by antigenic drift, combined with the inability of antibody produced by the host to eliminate the virus from the circulation, have rendered ineffective all attempts to produce vaccines to prevent lentivirus diseases in animals. Effective protection against infection with the AIDS virus using existing vaccination techniques would seem to be theoretically impossible.

Although other primates (e.g. monkeys) can be infected with HIV_1, they do not become ill in the absence of inducible illness, the protective effect of vaccine cannot be assessed in nonhuman animal models. But vaccine trials with humans will only cloud testing of blood donors since it will not be possible to distinguish between those with antibodies induced by vaccine since those vaccinated cannot be deliberately exposed to the virus to Judge their potential immunity to a lethal virus in view of the lack of protection so apparent from naturally induced antibodies

Unfortunately, a cure for *AIDS* will likely prove more elusive than an effective vaccine. According to Dr William O. Connor of Northern California; *any containment strategy upon the eventuality of a cure (for AIDS) is delusional. Once a retro virus has altered the genome (genes) of the host, if retain the ability to reproduce for the lifetime of the infected human.*

This is a consequence of the unique mechanism whereby RNA viruses infect their host. During the process of infection, the *AIDS* virus induces the production of a genetic fragment, its DNA biochemical mirror image as noted elsewhere, it's genetic particle insinuates itself into genetic substance of the host indefinitely.

This *AIDS* gene (termed proviral DNA) is therapeutically indistinguishable from the host genetic material. A successful medical regimen must selectively identify and destroy those specific virally induced sequences of DNA while maintaining the integrity of the host's genetic fabric. This goal is quite challenging but not insurmountable. Sequel to this the possibility exists for downgrading of AIDS from acute terminal disease to a chronic disease like diabetes or hypertension.

CHAPTER 9

COMMON SEXUALLY TRANSMITTED INFECTION (STI).

Many people are ignorant of sexually transmitted infection which can be passed from one person to another primarily by sexual contact or intercourse. Some of these infections do not show early clinical manifestation hence sexual partners can be infected and, in some cases, their unborn children. If untreated these infections can cause debilitating pain and destroys a girl's or woman's ability to have children. The mode of transmission is by infections agents like microscopic bacteria, viruses, parasite and single celled organisms like protozoa which can thrive in warm, moist environment in the body such as genital area, mouth and throat. Most sexually transmitted infections are spread during sexual intercourse (vagina, anal) but other forms of sexual contact, such as oral sex can also spread the infection. The infection can get into the baby as the baby passes through the birth canal. Common sexually transmitted infections are:

1.   CHLAMYDIA

This is caused by *chlamydia trachomatis*, may not produce noticeable symptoms, at often times it goes undiagnosed and the center for disease control estimate that the true incidence of chlamydia is nearly ten times the number of reported cases of those who do not know they are infected. Many may not seek medical care and may continue to infect other unknowingly spreading the disease. When symptoms do develop, boys may experience painful or burning urination, vagina discharge or mild lower abdominal pain in girls. If left untreated, chlamydia damages reproductive tissues causing inflammation of the urethra in male   (urethritis)   and   possibly   pelvic inflammatory disease can (PID) in female. Pelvic inflammatory disease can cause debilitating pelvic pain, infertility or fatal pregnancy complications. Chlamydia infection is diagnosed by testing penile and vaginal discharge for the presence of the bacteria.

2. GONORRHOEA.

This is caused by Neisseria gonorrhea or Gonococcus, it infects the membrane living cells of the genital. Male are more likely to develop symptoms that may be like those of chlamydia, include burning urination, penile or vagina discharge. Untreated gonorrhea can cause pelvic inflammatory disease (PID) in female, also salpingitis (which blocks the fallopian tube resulting in secondary infertility) Babies born to mother with gonorrhea can have eye disease (ophthalmia neonatorum). Gonorrhea is diagnosed by testing penile or vagina discharge specimen for the presence of

Neisseria gonorrhea. Typically, male symptoms are pain on passing urine, yellowish discharge from the penis. Delayed treatment can cause secondary infertility in male.

In female symptoms are increased vagina discharge, frequent or painful urination, high temperature and lower abdominal pain. If not treated timely the fallopian tube may be permanently blocked (salpingitis) and the female may never be able to have a baby.

3.   SYPHILIS

Is a potentially life threatening sexually transmitted infection caused by *treponema pallidum*. In the early stage of syphilis, a genital sore called *chancre* developed shortly after infection and eventually disappears on it own. If the disease is not treated, the infection can progress affecting the vertebrate, brain and heart resulting in such varied disorder as lack of co-ordination, meningitis and stroke. The symptoms are the same for male and female. During pregnancy, it can be devastating to the fetus causing deformity and death, but the good news is that it can be treated before the fetus is harmed.

4.   GENITAL WARTS.

This is transmitted by the human papillioma virus during sexual contact; grow on the penis and in or around the entrance to the vagina and anus. Although thay are relatively painless, genital warts can increase the risk of cancer of the cervix in female.

5.   TRICHOMONAL INFECTION

This is a common infection due to *trichomonas virginalis* which is yellow and has a noticeable smell. It also causes the vagina to be red burning, itching, and discomfort. A female cannot be infected on contact with infected cloths or object but commonly by sexual intercourse. In male, trichomonas may cause urethritis.

6. PRURITIC INFECTION

Vaginal itching (Volvo-vagina pruritus), burning sensation upon urination and unusual discharge do not always mean one has a venereal disease, it could well mean a vaginal infection due to vaginal candidiasis.

7. GENITAL HERPES

This is caused by infection with herpes simplex virus (HSV), which infects the genital, and most of the genitals herpes are due to HSV type 2. It causes recurrent out breaks of painful sore or blisters on the genitals, although the disease often remain dormant without symptoms for long periods. In males it appears as small sore or blisters on the penis probably burning feeling when urinating. In female the blisters may be around the vaginal or in the cervix, with fever or headache the symptoms usually show two or twenty days after contact, without treatment the symptoms disappear in a week or two but may flare up latter.

PREVENTION OF SEXUALLY TRANSMITTED INFECTION

1.   Abstinence which means restraining from premarital and extramarital sex

2.   Early diagnosis prompt treatment.

CHAPTER 10

HIV/AIDS PREVENTION AMONG YOUNG PEOPLE

According special priority to young people will change the future course of the epidemic. Changing behaviors and expectations early results in life time of benefit both in HIV prevention and in overcoming HIV-related stigma. The challenge is to promote effective programs that engage young people in all aspects of the response to HIV/AIDS. In every country where HIV transmission has been reduced it has been among young people that the most spectacular reductions have occurred. - Peter Piot , Former Executive Director, UNAIDS.

The way to halt the spread of *HIV/AIDS* is to focus on young people, they are at the center of the global *HIV/AIDS* pandemic. They also are the world's greatest hope in the struggle against this fatal disease.

Basic HIV/AIDS Education

Ignorance and misinformation is very common among young people in Sub-Saharan Africa there by fuelling the AIDS pandemic. Basic HIV/AIDS education in a clear and precise format and template should be made mandatory and delivered to young people (aged 15-24) in absorbable bits. It's imperative the information significantly highlight risking sexual behaviours and how to overcome them. However, some believed that early education of young people about sexual integrity will promote promiscuity and premature sexual behaviour; and increase abortion and teenage pregnancy. But on the contrary, there are evidence that showed that comprehensive HIV/AIDS education leads to decline in infection rate.

Encourage Abstinence

In this age of sex and hypersexualised world, abstinence is seen as obsolete and crude method but it's imperative we have to empowered young people to abstain from sex until marriage, Schools should form abstinence-only clubs to support and empower young people with comprehensive sex education that is focussed on abstinence teaching them skills of how to delay onset of sexual intercourse until marriage, improving their negotiation skills so that they can negotiate from position of sound and adequate knowledge thereby not trading their sexual integrity for cash or kind. Unfortunately, the current trend showed increase rate of premarital sex stemming from cohabitation and excessive glamorisation of sex and sexual act.

Involving young people

Young people with integrity and moral uprightness should be used as role model for others to follow and should be included in HIV/AIDS conferences, workshops or seminars. Young people need safe and supporting environment to use their skills and potential in music, arts or craft to propagate impactful HIV campaign to positively influence fellow young people. In addition, respecting young people positive culture and modus operandi are likely to give government and organization easy access to young people to influence them significantly.

Discouraging substance abuse

Substance and drug abuse should be discouraged in young people because when they indulged in these, it distorts and negatively influence their decision especially in sexual mater and can lead to rape, sexual violence and protected sexual practice fuelling HIV sexual transmission.

Encouraging young people with HIV to share their story

Encouraging and supporting young people to share their struggles and victories in living with HIV/AIDS. This has two-way advantage, first it will reinforce information to produce and foster healthy habits against HIV/AIDS. Also, it will encourage people living with HIV to end stigma and the discrimination by coming out boldly to challenge these.

A-Z OF HIV/AIDS PREVENTION

A   Abstain from premarital sex

B   Be faithful to your partner

C   Collaborate with government and agencies.

D   Don't use blood contaminated sharp object

E Exercise maximum control over your sexual desire

F Fill you with information about the disease

G Get to know your HIV status

H Help one another to stop the transmission

I inquire more about mode of transmission

J Join forces with your community to stop the transmission

K Know the importance of abstinence

L Live your dream, avoid the virus

M Maintain sexual integrity

N No to premarital sex

O Organize consistent programmed about *HIV/AIDS*

P Promote young people campaign against *HIV/AIDS*

Q Quit Extramarital affairs

R Reach out to young people at risk

S Safe and supportive environment to avoid transmission

T Teach young people about dangers of premarital sex

U Understand your *HIV* status and takes responsibility

V Voluntary and confidential *HIV* counseling and testing

W Women who are pregnant be screened

X X-rated movies and other pornographic materials avoided.

Y Yield to precautionary measures.

Z Zip up

OUR RESPONSIBILITY.

1. Media campaign to your village, street, church etc. about *HIV/AIDS*. Delay can lead to infection. Speak to little groups of people or at least your own relative.

2. Study the facts about AIDS in literature which you can learn and pass it to others to deepen their knowledge.

3. Remember those who cannot read, share knowledge with them.

4. Avoid sexual intercourse before marriage and encourage others in same way. Young people have far greater chances of normal, physical and emotional developments if they do not have sexual intercourse before marriage.

5. Be faithful to your spouse.

6. Do not deprive young people knowledge and information about reproductive health

7. Parents are the best teacher.

8. Give them enough information according to their age.

9. Warn your girls about the dangers of sugar daddies.

10. Help young girls/women about the danger of trial marriage.

11. Encourage those that have been infected.

12. Do not take injection anyhow, go to a good hospital.

13. Ensured blood products screened before transfusion.

CHAPTER 11

LEGAL APPROACHES TO HIV/AIDS

We live in a time of madness, a time when public and private foolishness reigns we have among us a plague, a disease so deadly that anyone who is contaminated will likely die... In California, the madness is complete. A doctor is restricted by law from informing another doctor that a referred patient had AIDS (in infection). Legally, doctor cannot tell hospital nurses or any health care provider who may come in contact with the infected person, that his patient has AIDS (infection). Doctor can't even inform the spouse of an infected individual. What monumental ignorance, what dangerous superciliousness, what deadly logic; murder in the name of privacy.

-Sen. H.L Richardson, California state Assembly, Aug. 1987.

Society will in some manner likely solve the *AIDS* dilemma, but in the meantime, solving this will take some adroit doing. The government is empowered to act in response to a health hazard at both federal and state levels. Any such action must be narrowly directed at control of the viral infection and be devoid of personal prejudicial motives.

With this consideration in mid, it must be understood that in order to eliminate *AIDS*, it is necessary to identify it (that is the infected reservoir) and then interrupt its known means of spread.

Identification will necessitate mandatory national serologic testing while interdictions of spread will require behavioral change.
Where such change is not voluntarily undertaken, statuary restraints must be enacted to selectively restrict individual

behavior to the degree necessary, relying on knowledge of the specific modes of transmission.

The federal government should be empowered to prevent spread of disease across state or national border through a mandatory national blood testing for individual. The identity of all the sero positive individual should then be entered in a national repository and confidentially maintained under the aegis of specifically designated treatment centers.

Measures should be drawn at the state level to vigorously discourage and interrupts continued *AIDS* transmission as follows. Here are some thoughtful suggestions.

1. Define *AIDS* as a communicable contagious disease commencing at the time of infection and require all sero positive case to be reported to the designated state health centers as is the

current practice for other dangerous, communicable disease and standard contact tracing procedure should follow every reported case.

2. Empower physicians to obtain *HIV* blood test on all patients in whom they deem it medically necessary

3. Initiate mandatory *HIV* testing of all hospital admitter between the age of 15 and 55.

4. Institute serologic screening of patient at sexually transmitted infection (STI) clinics

5. Require mandatory *HIV* testing for marital license applicants

6. Provide criminal penalty for anyone donating blood who is a member of a high-risk group like homosexual, drug abuser, commercial sex worker.

7. Activate existing quarantine measures to selectively restrict the activity of

those infected individuals whose continued irresponsible or incompetent conduct is likely to further propagate infection. The result of this will lead to elimination of *AIDS* as a competitor with human kind for species survival before the epidermis matches irrevocably beyond society's grasp.

LAST WORD

THE DEFEAT OF AIDS

Flee fornication (those not married should abstain from sexual intercourse) - 1 Corinthians 6:18

AIDS differs from some other epidemics in one important aspect; it is preventable if young people and individuals are prepared to adhere to basic Bible principles and precepts, they can in many of not all cases avoid contamination.

The bible moral codes are clear, the unmarried should abstained from sexual intercourse (1 Corinthians 6:18), married ones should be faithful to their partners and abstain from extra marital sex (Hebrew 13:4).

Health professionals must aptly point out that behavioral changes as a vital strategy in defeat of *AIDS. Each generation of young people* says a report published by the Center for Disease Control and Prevention *needs comprehensive, sustained health information and intervention that help them develop lifelong skills for avoiding behaviors that could lead to HIV infection. Such comprehensive program includes the involvement of parent as well as educators.*

Clearly, parents need to educate their children about these dangers before their peers corrupt them. This is not an easy task. But it can save your child's life and present a generation from damage. Informing children about sexuality need not take away innocence but protect them from losing it. Among God's ancient people, parents were expected to teach their children about sexuality and how to protect their health.

Interestingly the Bible provides us with clear moral guidelines and signposts for protection from diseases for example.

How are these principles to be taught? Parent first had to understand the benefits of adherence and the consequence for negligence *Deuteronomy 6:6-7 And these words which I command you today shall be in your heart. You shall teach them diligently to your children and shall talk of them when you sit in your house, when you walk by the way, when you lie down, and when you rise up.*

This means to teach and impress by frequent repetition or admonitions, obviously time is involved. Parents who set aside time to teach their sons and daughters about dangers of illicit sex stand a better chance of seeing their children avoid types of behavior that can lead to contracting *HIV* and other disease.

BIBLOGRAPHY

1. HIV and Young People, Joint United National Program on HIV/AIDS and WHO, 2002.
2. The Nation's First Politically Protected Disease AIDS. Mcnamee JL, California 1988.

www.ingramcontent.com/pod-product-compliance
Lightning Source LLC
Chambersburg PA
CBHW072047230526
45468CB00019B/496